How To

Increase

Testosterone

Naturally

The How &

Why Of

Getting High Levels Of Testosterone Naturally

Charles Sledge

Table Of Contents

Introduction

Across the Western world there has been a decline in masculinity. Some say this decline has been engineered while others say it has come about because of changing lifestyle. Regardless of the reason the problem is still here and is having negative effects all across society.

The root of this problem is because of a decline in the testosterone levels of men. Nearly everything in the modern world is geared toward lowering one's testosterone levels and making him less of a man in the process.

A war has been waged on your hormones and for too long it has gone unanswered. But no more. This book will give you to tools that you need to fight back and regain hormonal health and balance. And increase your testosterone levels beyond what they have ever been before.

This book is for men of all ages. From boys entering puberty in a world filled with anti-masculine forces and chemicals to a man in his eighties wanting to stay a man until his final days.

Many of the issues plaguing modern males can be traced back to lack of masculinity which has a direct correlation with a lack of testosterone. Testosterone is the elixir of life which is why it is demonized and attacked by the main stream. Testosterone makes men out of boys and free men out of slaves.

A population with high levels of testosterone is not easy to control or to lead astray. As a man testosterone is one of the most precious assets that you have, it is your life blood. And is it being taken from you every day.

From the stuff that is put in the water, to the mindset the modern world would have you adapt, to one hundred other things. There is a war on your masculinity and the greatest battle in that war is the battle for your testosterone.

We live in a world and society when even teenagers are suffering from low levels of testosterone. Many having the testosterone levels of the "average" eighty year old man. And yet nothing is said of this or it is brushed off as the "new normal".

This is an abomination. Perhaps all you wish for is an increased sex drive or higher energy levels and that is why you picked up this book. You will get all of that and so much more when you follow what is lain out here.

Regardless of what brought you here prepare for your life to be changed with the knowledge in this book. I don't say this as some feel good self-help nonsense but as a biological reality.

The higher your testosterone is the more of a man you are and the more of a man that you are the better and greater life that you will lead.

But enough about what is to be. Now it is time to learn the steps to take to raise your testosterone as high as it can be naturally. I do not talk about TRT (testosterone replacement therapy) in this book and if finding that after doing everything here (especially for men over 50) that you still don't feel vigorous and strong then that is an option you may want to consider.

Regardless it is wise to learn all that you can of this life giving hormone, this lifeblood of man so that you can get all that you can out of life.

Now go and be a man.

The Many Positive Effects Of Having High Levels Of Testosterone

Testosterone is perhaps the most important hormone when it comes to a man's enjoyment of life and his masculinity. This hormone is responsible for the vast majority of what makes a man a man. Guys who go from having low levels of testosterone to having high levels of testosterone feel like completely new men. They feel completely reborn and one hundred times the man that they used to be.

Testosterone is the elixir of life and that's not exaggeration. The more testosterone that a man has the better off that he'll be, plain and simple. Here I'm going to expand on some of the many benefits of increasing your testosterone.

These benefits extend from how masculine you feel, to the bedroom, to work, to play, to intelligence, to earning potential, to quality of life, to just about everything else. The more you increase your testosterone the better off you are in pretty much every facet of your life. Men with high testosterone do and accomplish more. After all it's the elixir of life. I'm not going to be able to cover everything here as an entire book could be written about the positive effects of having high testosterone but I'm going to hit on some key points that are guaranteed to have an impact on your life. Alright let's get started.

Increased Sex Drive

And that's putting it lightly. Testosterone is the number one determinant in how horny a human being is. The higher the testosterone the higher the sex drive. Believe it or not but in my experience many males trouble with women doesn't stem from not having "game" (though that can be a factor) but rather from not having a high enough sex drive. This stems from having low testosterone as well as their dopamine being screwed up by watching and masturbating to porn so much. Combine the two and you have the perfect storm of screwed up sexuality and sexual desire.

When you have high testosterone you are always on the lookout for sex. This isn't a uncontrollable lust like you'd have for something that messed with your dopamine (such as drugs and porn) but rather something that is much healthier feeling and under your control. Higher testosterone is also a cause of harder and bigger erections which is certainly a bonus. Not only will you want sex more but you will be prepared for it more. A guy with high testosterone is ready to go all the time. Having higher testosterone also helps you last longer in the bedroom. So higher sex drive, better sex, and overall better feelings.

Fat Loss & Muscle Gain

Trying to get someone to grow muscles without having high testosterone levels is like trying to plant a flower in the desert. It's going to be hard work for mediocre gains. Likewise having high testosterone is like placing that same flower in the Garden of Eden mixed with super grow. It's going to grow like crazy. Instead of working even harder at the gym (with less and less to show for it) your lack of gains (or loss) might be from having low levels of testosterone. If you're having trouble gaining muscle (and you're working out, eating right, and sleeping well) then it's most likely because you have low levels of testosterone.

Testosterone makes losing fat and gaining muscle a whole lot easier. Like I said it's like the difference between planting a flower in the desert and planting a flower in the Garden of Eden. It's a night and day difference. This is one of the primary reasons why as a man ages a certain amount it gets harder and harder to lose fat and put on muscle. How many guys work twice as hard as they did when they were in their twenties yet have far less to show for it? Get your testosterone levels right and you don't have to worry about that nearly as much. Testosterone will do wonders for your body composition.

Energy & Mind

The mainstream media would like you to believe (among other things) that testosterone is evil and will turn you into an angry maniac when the fact of the matter is testosterone is going to do the opposite. Testosterone improves your mood and increases your feelings of well-being. Not to mention that testosterone also increases the clarity of thought and how sharp your mind is. Here's how I would describe it. Have you ever been dead tired and dehydrated and sat down to work on something. Say write an article, chapter, or report? Your mind is scrambled and it's hard to get coherent thoughts together.

So you get some sleep and drink lots of water. Then the ideas and what you want just flow out of you and onto the paper. That's the difference between your mind with low testosterone and high testosterone. Testosterone is also correlated with energy. Meaning the more testosterone you have the more energy that you are going to have. And I'm not talking about hyper jittery energy like you get from caffeine and stimulants but rather a strong controlled energy. A healthy energy (sort of like the difference between dopamine high seeking horniness and testosterone horniness, one's unhealthy and feels bad the other is healthy and feels good). Again another reason why younger males tend to have higher energy levels than older males.

Summary

These are just some of the many benefits of having healthy testosterone levels. And chances are if you are a male living in the Western world you are suffering from lower levels of testosterone than you should and therefore are missing out on all these great benefits as well as feeling like more of a man and having a higher quality of life. Want to get laid more then get your testosterone up. Want to look better then get your testosterone up. Want to feel better and thinker better then get your testosterone up. Want to feel like more of a man? Well you know what to do. Testosterone is the elixir of life and it's always in your best interest to maximize it.

3 Ways To Raise Your Testosterone Naturally

Alright so if you're a man then you know that testosterone in particular having high testosterone is one of the most important factors for determining the quality of your life as well as how good you feel as a man. With low testosterone levels you're just not going to feel like yourself, although with younger generations they may very well go their entire lives without knowing what having proper testosterone levels feels like. Regardless the higher your testosterone the better that you will feel and the better quality of life that you will have. If you're an average male living in Western society then chances are your testosterone levels are lacking.

Before looking at different measures to increase your testosterone the first thing that you are going to want to do is make sure that you have the basics covered. Meaning that before you look into what type of TRT you want to go on or other methods you want to make sure you are doing all that you can naturally for added effect in addition to overall good health. Not to mention that everything laid out here is going to be good for other health factors in your life as well. Testosterone is very much a sign of an overall healthy male body. Though there are certain things that can be done to specifically increase testosterone as well. Just like you can tailor an overall nutrition program and workout program for bigger arms or chiseled abs you can do the same for high testosterone (which will do a hundred times more for you than anything else you can tailor it for).

Sleeping For Testosterone

Sleep is incredibly important for a number of factors. It is during sleep that your body rebuilds and recharges from the day. In particular what is important is deep sleep or

REM sleep. Testosterone levels tend to rise the longer that one is asleep and REM sleep has a particularly strong effect on this. The longer you sleep the better off you'll be. For both testosterone levels and muscle repair and growth. Sure it might be trendy and you'll impress your hipster friends if you cut your sleep into short blocks to "get more done" or whatever but your testosterone levels are also going to take a dive.

My advice would be if you really need to get more done then just work harder during the day like a normal human being. Don't mess with your sleep. You want to get at least eight hours a night. Sure there are some people who can do "okay" with a little less but two things. One you're probably not one of them if you're active and two who the hell wants to just be "okay"? You want to make sure your sleep is long and uninterrupted. Use the bathroom before bed, make sure there are no lights in the bedroom, make sure your shades are drawn, use a sleep mask and relaxing music if you have to, and make sure your bedroom is cool. Sleep is critical to healthy testosterone production. Again make sure it's deep, long, and uninterrupted for maximum effect.

Eating For Testosterone

Not all diets are created equal neither are all calories despite the delusion of many a fitness trainer and scientist that they are. Alright first things first if you're eating for testosterone you can throw out pretty much any form of mainstream diet. Two in particular that are guaranteed to destroy your testosterone levels are low fat diets and vegan diets. Two diets that also seem to be pushed a lot. Look if you want to be weak, pasty, doughy, and a pussy then vegan and low fat diets are perfect however if you want to be a strong man then you're going to have to eat very differently. In particular you are going to want to eat plenty of good fats.

What are the good fats? Well essentially all fats that occur naturally, in particular saturated fat. The kind that is on red meats, eggs, and that our best buddies who have our best interest at heart at the government have told us to avoid for so long. If you want good levels of testosterone then you are going to have to eat good amounts of good fats, saturated fats in particular. So be sure to break out the bacon and whole eggs for breakfast and the steak for dinner. Fats are essential for hormone optimization and making sure that everything is running properly. Especially testosterone production. So make sure to get in a good amount of fats.

Lifting For Testosterone

Alright to optimize testosterone production in the gym you want to make sure to only do isolation exercises and run long distance. After all look at marathon runners they're the peak of human development and what's more manly than them? Alright I'm kidding but I think you see where I'm going with this. We all know the lifts that are going to increase our testosterone. Full body lifts that are tried and true. Things like squatting, pressing, and deadlifting. Also sprints work great as well. You want to make sure you're getting adequate volume as well. You don't have to go all

German Volume Training but at least Reg Park's 5×5.

You want to lift heavy weights for adequate volume, let's put it like that. Full body training, barbell complexes, and sprints are all great ways to train for optimum testosterone production. Use big compound movements that require effort and really get you going. Ass to grass squats are going to do a lot more for your testosterone production then isolation curls (plus they probably going to do more for your bicep as well). Stick to squats, deadlifts, presses, rows, pullups, and Olympic movements for your workout. Save the isolation work for the end if it's even needed. You also might want to add in some barbell complexes or sprints at the end of your workout for extra testosterone production and fat loss.

Summary

There is nothing revolutionary here, it's all pretty basic. But the basics are fundamental to success. Before you move on you have to master the basics. If you're not doing the above things already then you shouldn't be complaining about low testosterone levels. Get these things right and then worry about other stuff. If you're not already doing these things then start. They'll have a huge impact on how you feel and how masculine you are. I can think of few better reasons to take one's health matters into their own hands then a better quality of life and optimal testosterone production.

80% Of Game Is Having High Testosterone

Alright so pretty much everyone knows that there is a correlation between testosterone levels and sex drive. How deep and important the correlation is may be a mystery many but most understand that there is at least a connection. However what most do not understand is that the vast majority of issues that modern males have with women (in particular not having the sex life they want with the women they want) stems from having low levels of testosterone. Sure other things play a role but nothing plays as important or as large of a role as testosterone. No dating coach will tell you this (as it would destroy his business model) but it's the truth.

There is a war on masculinity (and therefore testosterone). There could be (and is) multiple books written on the subject. Because of this many males today have never had healthy proper testosterone levels. It has be struck out of them from a variety of sources. From the schools, to the media, to the government, and more. Testosterone levels have been plummeting for the last 25 years (and longer than that). The average male does not have the same level of testosterone that his father had at his age and certainly not his grandfather. This leads to a whole host of negative effects throughout society. Here we are going to address men not having the sex life that they want.

The "Natural"

The concept of a "dating coach" would be completely foreign to my father and grandfather and was completely foreign to me for the longest time. A boxing coach sure, a sales trainer alright, even a nutritionist getting a little out there but whatever, but a dating coach? To men with high testosterone a dating coach would be like having a coach to use the restroom or swallow your food. Something that is done naturally and not something you put any thought into. What dating coaches call "naturals" are simply guys with high testosterone. Simple as that. Guys with high testosterone never think about lines or techniques, they simply are and women are attracted to them.

It's natural. How it was always supposed to be. Women are attracted to testosterone. They want manly masculine men meaning men with high testosterone. To get the sex life he wants with the women he wants a guy would be better off raising his testosterone then he would getting on any dating program or with any dating coach in the world. Success with women stems from masculinity, success with women stems from testosterone. The sooner a guy gets this the better off he'll be. Many males spend a good chunk of their life chasing after women with a myriad of different techniques and theories but they get him little to no success. Only masculinity and testosterone will get him what he wants in that area of his life.

Libido & Testosterone

Your libido and sex drive is directly correlated to how high your testosterone is. Look at it like this the guys who sleep with the most women are the guys with the highest levels of testosterone plain and simple. The higher your testosterone the more you want sex, the more you want sex the more you'll go out and get it. If you want something more you'll go after it more. The guy who has to pee five times a day is going to go to the rest room more than the guy who has to pee once a day. Doesn't matter how close each guy is to the bathroom or what kind of bathroom they use. Guys with higher testosterone are going to have more sex, more frequently than guys with high testosterone.

Take a guy with great "game" but with average testosterone levels and put him against a guy who has no idea what "game" is but has high testosterone levels. And the guy with higher testosterone levels is going to sleep with more women at the end of the month every time. Trying to get good at game or dating is a hamster wheel. It's like pressing on the accelerator harder and harder or changing out tires when the car doesn't even have an engine. The more you have testosterone the more you're going to get after it (and actually get it) so if you're one of those guys who's not having the success with women he wants. Drop the dating coach and learn how to increase your testosterone.

How To Be In The Top Tier Of Guys

There is a sexual pyramid if you will. Meaning that there are guys at the top and guys at the bottom. The men at the top are the twenty percent of guys that sleep with eighty percent of women. The males at the bottom are the eighty percent of guys who settle for the twenty percent scraps that the top guys didn't want. It's not fair but it is life. The main thing that separates the guys at the top from the guys at the bottom is their testosterone levels. The guys at the top are the guys with high testosterone levels and the guys at the bottom are the guys with low testosterone levels.

There are different ways to get into the top but the absolute best and quickest way is to get your testosterone levels up. Eighty percent of "game" or whatever you want to call it (sexual success with women) is having high levels of testosterone. Not memorizing complex theories, not having a harmonious inner self, not lines, not anything but having high levels of testosterone (being a man). That's it. The more people that find this out the better off everyone will be (except those who make their living pushing products on picking up women and such).

Summary

This is the Pareto principle when applies to sexual success with women. Sure things like mindset and others things certainly have value and they matter but they are the eighty percent of effort that gets you twenty percent of results. It's the high testosterone levels that are the twenty percent of effort that are going to give you eighty percent of results. Not to mention testosterone has tons of other benefits far beyond your dating and sex life. Get this right and many other things will fall into place. Remember be a man and

everything else will fall into place.
Your sex life is no exception.

How To Boost Testosterone Through Supplementation

Let me start off my saying as a whole I'm not a big fan of supplements. Most are overhyped and as effective as sugar pills in getting what you want out of them. For the most part unless you're looking for great marketing stay away from supplements. However with that being said there are some exceptions. Also something to keep in mind is what the entire point of supplements are (or at least are supposed to be). Supplements despite many marketing claims to the contrary are not magical pills. There is no pill that you'll take where you'll end up big and ripped just because you took it.

Supplements are supposed to be supplemental to a well-balanced nutritious diet. You would think that would be self-explanatory from the name but it's not. Many see supplements as the main key to getting what they want instead of lifting, nutrition, and recovery which are the true keys to getting what you want. Where supplements come in handy is when they address an imbalance or a lack of something that you aren't getting in your diet. For example say you're eating fish every day then throwing in a fish oil supplement (one supplement I actually overall recommend) isn't going to do much for you. However if you're getting in little to no omega 3's to balance out your omega 6's then supplementing with fish oil could have dramatic changes.

Testosterone Boosters

Alright so let's start off with the natural choice, testosterone boosters. Testosterone boosters are naturally what most people go to when they are looking to raise their testosterone levels. After all it's right there in the name. Unfortunately test boosters (unless they're a prohormone or steroid) are completely useless. Anything that you can get over the counter from your local supplement store isn't going to do much of anything to raise your testosterone levels (though it will do a great job of making your wallet lighter). These "testosterone boosters" are really just high priced junk that's marketed very well.

Natural test boosters supplements should be avoided. They aren't going to do anything for you. I know the ripped guy on the cover says it's how he got his body (had nothing to do with the real steroids of course) and there's a study in the ad that says it boosts testosterone 1,000% and as we know studies can be trusted one hundred percent and completely replace our need for rational thought, just kidding. But you get the point. There is a way to boost testosterone through supplementation but it has nothing to do with natural test boosters. It has to do with addressing deficiencies in vitamins and minerals that lead to testosterone production. So throw out the test boosters and save your money for something that'll actually make a difference.

ZMA

I originally started taking ZMA back in college to help me sleep. I was having trouble going to bed sometimes and didn't necessarily like melatonin except for if I really had to get to bed. So I was recommended ZMA because it was said to help me sleep. I'm not sure how much of an effect ZMA has on sleep but I do know that it has an impact on other things. Namely sex drive and erection strength. Turns out both two of the minerals contained in ZMA, zinc and magnesium are very important when it comes to testosterone production and are deficient in many males even those who have a relatively healthy diet. I had been eating good but was still lacking this vital minerals that were able to give me that extra edge.

Zinc alone is amazing in all the benefits that it has for men. Factor in magnesium as well and you have a supplement that can actually make a difference when it comes to testosterone production. There is a correlation between having adequate zinc intake and testosterone levels as well as a correlation between having adequate magnesium levels and testosterone levels. Not to mention the added sleep benefit isn't going to hurt either (putting it lightly) making ZMA a great supplement for men who want to make sure they are producing as much testosterone as possible. And let's be honest what type of man doesn't want that?

Vitamin D

Are you getting at least an hour or so of sun a day? If not then you're deficient in this essential hormone. That's right hormone. "Vitamin" D is actually a hormone and very important in the production of testosterone. Most of us (even those of us living in year round sunny areas) do not get enough sun. We spend too much time indoors and most of us work away our days in an office and then return home once the sun has gone down. Even those of us who don't spend our days in an office still probably aren't getting as much sun as we should and therefore not getting adequate vitamin D.

Factor in areas where for a good five months out of the year there is little to no sun and it's almost a guarantee that you (and your testosterone levels) will benefit from supplementing with vitamin D. Those with vitamin D deficiencies found that after supplementing with vitamin D for a year raised their testosterone levels by 25% from the vitamin D alone. Perhaps a year seems like a long time but you'd be missing the bigger picture if that's what you're focusing on. 25% is one hell of an increase especially from one little supplement (a hell of a lot more than any over the counter "test booster" will get you). So be sure to supplement with vitamin D it's both cheap and effective.

Summary

Remember at the end of the day these are all just supplements. They are made to address common deficiencies and that's it. They aren't made to replace working out properly, getting enough sleep, or eating the right foods. They are supplements meaning that they are supplemental. They can certainly give you an edge and help with testosterone production but don't focus on them and ignore everything else as many tend to do. Use the above supplements you can find them cheap online or at your local store. Both of them together will cost less than one bottle of worthless test booster anyways.

How To Decrease Your Estrogen

If you're looking to maximize your testosterone and feel like more of a man then not only do you need to focus on testosterone optimization but everything that goes along with testosterone. Testosterone does not exist in a vacuum meaning that there are many other things that affect it. For example someone could have very high levels of total testosterone yet still not get the many positive effects of it because of he has very low levels of free testosterone. Meaning testosterone that hasn't been binded and is freely availble for us by the body. So in order to optimize free testosterone and get all of the positive effects associated with it one must also take care of other issues as well in addition to maximizing total testosterone levels.

A prime example of this is a man's estrogen levels. Now a man will naturally have some low levels of estrogen which is good and healthy however it becomes a problem when his estrogen levels get too high (as in the case of the majority of modern males) this can happen because one's testosterone levels raise suddenly and drastically (such as when injecting testosterone) and can also happen from other negative things that raise your estrogen levels above where they should naturally be at. You must take steps in order to ensure that you are keeping your estrogen levels down so that your testosterone can be increased and has the best chances of becoming free testosterone which is what gives you all the positive effects associated with testosterone.

Lose The Fat

Notice that I didn't say lose the weight. But specifically lose the fat, getting rid of fat (especially stomach fat) is going to help decrease over all estrogen levels in your body and thereby allow for more free testosterone. There is a direct correlation with how much fat that a man has and how high his estrogen levels are. Meaning the fatter that a man is the more estrogen that his body has. Get rid of the fat and you'll get rid of a good portion of the bad estrogen. Losing weight alone doesn't mean anything, it's losing fat specifically. Especially fat that is centered around your waist in men.

Estrogen and fat cells go together like peanut butter and jelly. And fat cells and testosterone go together like oil and water. The less fat a guy has is correlated directly with higher levels of testosterone. Note that a guy could be big and still have high testosterone based on a variety of factors but fat (especially gut fat) does a guy no favors. Likewise one could be a twig with a bit of a gut and have high levels of estrogen. Get rid of fat and build muscle, it's as simple as that. The best way to get rid of fat and thereby lower estrogen is one by good dieting and two by doing intense cardio such as barbell complexes, sprints, or Tabata workouts.

Watch Out For Chemicals

There are chemicals everywhere and I literally mean everywhere. From the water that you drink to the foods that you eat. There are unnatural chemicals that mess with your body and your sensitive endocrine system (which largely controls your testosterone production). These chemicals can really screw us up and raise our estrogen levels, some are certainly worse than others but no matter what the less unnatural chemicals that you expose yourself to the better off you'll be and the lower your estrogen levels will be. I used to think this was all hype but it's very real and has a huge impact on your testosterone and estrogen levels.

Xenoestrogens and a host of other chemicals that mimic estrogen in the body (and therefore have the same effects) are contained in many different items we use every day. It would be like having an IV of estrogen slowly dripping into our system throughout the day, destroying our testosterone levels. Here are the biggest offenders to avoid. First off plastics. Don't drink out of plastic water bottles (perhaps the worst of plastics) and don't eat from plastic containers. You want to drink filtered water (as tap water is another key offender) from a non-plastic container. Don't keep refilling (or ever using in the first place) plastic water bottles. Get something else that is free of all those things.

Another thing to watch out for is many personal products especially if they contain parabens (if you see something listed paraben in the ingredients ditch it). Switch to more natural made stuff. Sure it might cost a little more but your hormonal health is well worth it trust me. Eat organic meats, meat is great when it's organic grass fed meat and not processed crap. Unfortunately processed meats contain many different hormones and estrogenic compound that'll raise your estrogen levels and destroy the value of any macronutrients. So make sure to eat grass fed organic meats. Also you want to watch out for anything containing BPA which has actually been shown to change male animals to female animals (you read that right). That's how estrogenic that crap is. Avoid it like the plague.

Cut Out Alcohol

What if I told you there was a substance that could all at the same time make you dumber, make you fatter, make your weaker, all while destroying your manhood, decreasing testosterone levels, skyrocketing estrogen levels, and ensuring that your dick didn't work how well do you think that product would sell? Well turns out pretty damn well. Alcohol (the woman maker as it should be referred to) does all of this and at incredibly high prices. Of course binge drinking is worse than lightly drinking but nevertheless you're always better off with water. Alcohol destroys testosterone levels and increases estrogen like crazy when consumed in large amounts. Drinking a lot also increases the rate at which testosterone in converted into estrogen.

The worst offender for alcohol is beer by a long shot. The hoppier the beer the worse that it is for you. If I were you I'd start calling beer by its real name estrogen shot because that is exactly what it is. Think about what the average guy does to his body every weekend when he pounds back estrogen shot after estrogen shot it's a wonder that males in the Western world have balls that actually work. Far from being a man drink this drink is actually the biggest woman maker out there. Avoid beer and alcohol especially drinking it in large amounts. Trust me with lower levels of estrogen and high testosterone you'll never have to worry about relying on alcohol to socialize, approach women, feel good, or get through the day. Testosterone provides all of that in spades.

Summary

To get all the positive effects of testosterone you have to look at more than just regular testosterone levels. You also have to take into account things like estrogen and other factors that might keep your testosterone from having it's intended effect on you. It's not enough to focus on simply testosterone alone, to have optimized free testosterone levels. Follow the steps outlined here to ensure that your estrogen is being kept in check and isn't destroying your levels of testosterone and keeping you from being a man. Make sure to get rid of that fat, especially if you have a gut (perhaps caused by beer?), avoid chemicals, and don't drink alcohol especially to excess. Do that and you'll help lower your estrogen levels and keep free testosterone high.

A Potent One Two Punch To Sky Rocket Your Libido

A man's sex drive is one of the most telling signs of his health in particular his hormonal health. We should be virile and manly throughout our entire lives. Not just in our twenties (and even now that is rapidly becoming an age when males have trouble with their libido). We were made to be vigorous and filled with testosterone and masculinity from puberty to the grave. So first off cast off any limiting beliefs of "Oh I'm age X and therefore can't do Y". For the most part they are bullshit. With hard work, determination, and knowledge you can reverse trends and defy what is in store for the "average" person. Your sex drive is very important, it's a sign of energy, health, and vitality.

Many may think that focusing on their sex drive is vain or not nearly as important as other things. Without realizing that their sex drive is a reflection of their overall health and in particular their hormonal health. If you are suffering from a low sex drive that is a sign that something is wrong and you are not living optimally. Remember you should always live with vigor and that masculine energy coursing through your veins. Here I'm going to show you a very potent one two punch that is sure to increase your libido and imbue your life with the masculine energy that gives it so much of its zest.

Raising Your Testosterone

Raising your testosterone is the number one thing that you can do to increase your libido. There is a war on testosterone it has been demonized as a hormone responsible for all of society's ills as well as for anger issues. When in fact testosterone is responsible for creating society and for controlling anger instead of lashing out like a low T little girl. Likewise now that those myths have been debunked new lies sprout up about how testosterone can lead to heart attacks or that testosterone actually doesn't increase your libido past a very small amount (laughable to anyone who has high testosterone or ever done a bottle of T). The doctors, media, and other liars of our time will do all they can to demonize and destroy this God given hormone.

From saying it's too powerful to saying it's not powerful at all. Testosterone and libido are directly correlated. There is no denying this. Raise your testosterone and you raise your libido. Simple as that. The more testosterone that you have the hornier you will get. Every man I know who sleeps with the most women or has the most vigorous sex life has high levels of testosterone. There is a reason that men want sex so much more than women, because of testosterone. This is why gay men can have over one thousand partners and lesbians won't even sleep with the one they have (check Kinsey research and lesbian bed death). Because of testosterone. Getting your testosterone up is the number one thing that you can do to increase your libido. The higher your T goes the higher your libido goes.

Cut Out Porn

Testosterone is not the only thing that plays a role in your libido (though it is certainly the primary and most important thing). Dopamine also plays a role as well, including how your brain is wired and what it responds to. Porn can really screw up how your brain works and especially your dopamine. Porn can make it so that you get more turned on by a flashing light of a computer screen than by real life flesh and blood. Not to mention that porn can also lead to ED and troubles with being attracted to women in real life. The trouble with your libido could be related to porn and in particular what porn does to your dopamine.

Dopamine plays a major role in arousal and going after the things that you want (such as good looking women). When your dopamine circuitry is messed up as well as you have numbed yourself through dopamine abuse (which porn and especially porn with masturbation will do) then you're going to have sexual issues and issues with your libido. Now I've seen guys with high testosterone cancel this out but nevertheless they'd be better off with just cutting out porn as well, which would increase their libido and desire for real women even more as well as get their dopamine functioning properly once again. So cut out porn to get a boost to your libido as well (it could take some time to get to normal functioning if you've been chronically using it for some time).

Your Libido

As with everything else things like diet, exercise, sleep, stress, and lifestyle are also going to play a big role (these things are all tied to hormonal health as well). So make sure that your hitting the gym and doing intense weight training or HIIT style cardio. No steady state T killing crap. Make sure that you're getting good sleep and sleeping for at least eight hours in a dark room. Keep stress as low as possible the biggest way to do this is to not worry about small stuff and to stay away from the news, meditation can also help with this as well. And finally you want a lifestyle that is conducive to good health. Obviously this is very broad but you can imagine it doesn't include boozing all night and doing drugs.

Speaking of which you want to make sure you're staying away from alcohol. Especially drinking heavily. A lot of this stuff is common sense and the wise have known what they are talking about for ages. There is a reason strong men from the 1800s knew eating eggs and doing squats was good for your body. Something that studies are just now starting to get around their head. True knowledge doesn't come from a test tube or nerds in lab coats. It comes from experience in the real world and seeing what works with your own eyes and the eyes of others. I see so many try to increase their libido and hormone health by reading study after study conducted on rats with inconclusive evidence that contradicts the ten other studies like it. See what works for you leave the studies for those who want to be two hundred plus years behind the times.

Summary

You were meant to live with health and vigor until the end of your days.

Don't listen to the doctors and media of today that do not have your best interest at heart or are fools. Man was made to live strong and virile until they put him in the ground. This can be possible for you barring any severe medical condition. You were meant to live with health in particular hormonal health. This starts with getting your testosterone levels up and then getting them higher and higher as well as cutting out things like porn that can screw up your dopamine and therefore sex drive. As well as living an overall healthy lifestyle. Now get to it.

Hormones & Raising Your Testosterone

In addition to doing everything possible to raise your actual total testosterone levels another thing you have to make sure of for optimal free testosterone levels (the kind the counts) is to make sure that your hormones are in balance and that you are doing everything possible to maximize the amount of total testosterone not only produced but also converted into free testosterone. There are many things that can get in the way of this and if not addressed can ruin your chances of having high free testosterone levels and all of the myriad of benefits that go along with that. No matter what the foundation of healthy testosterone levels (as well as overall hormonal balance) comes from a base of good health.

There are some hormones in particular that can get in the way of your free testosterone and that can destroy the amount of total testosterone converted into free testosterone. Most people never address these things when talking about raising testosterone and even recommend things that are detrimental to your overall hormonal health. That is what happens when you focus on rat studies instead of what actually happens in humans and using common sense. Here I'm going to talk about three key hormones and what you can do to ensure that they don't interfere with your free testosterone as well as debunk some myths that have been circulating around the raising testosterone community and are detrimental to progress.

Cortisol

Cortisol is known as the stress hormone. And obviously it's related to stress. To put it simply and so you can get the general idea of all of this is that the more stress that you have the more cortisol that you're going to have and that is bad for testosterone (especially free testosterone). Stress kills testosterone. It could be high levels of physical stress, say working long shifts day in and day out or from partying nonstop and not taking care of your health. It could be from work related stress such as a POS boss shafting you every chance he gets or a job that is naturally high stress and doesn't allow for much recuperation. Doesn't matter if it's physical or mental it still causes cortisol which will lower testosterone levels.

You want to make sure that you are keeping your cortisol levels low because the higher your cortisol is the lower your testosterone is going to be. They have a reverse effect on one another. So you want to make sure that you are avoiding overtraining (meaning stressing your body out too much with long training sessions). With the gym you want to get in and get out with high intensity. Likewise you want to avoid stress as much as possible. Do things like meditation, going for a walk in nature, or listening to classical music, these things all lower cortisol. And the number one thing for lowering cortisol (and perhaps total hormone health) is making sure that you get adequate deep sleep. Do everything you can to make sure your sleep in uninterrupted as well as deep. Deep sleep is a cortisol killer and incredible testosterone booster.

Aromatase

Alright so you know in order to have high levels of testosterone you know that you have to keep your estrogen levels down. Estrogen and testosterone are not going to go together. The lower you can get your estrogen the higher you can get your testosterone essentially. Now in particular something you want to make sure is regulated and taken care of is aromatase. Aromatase is an adrenal enzyme that converts potential testosterone into estrogen.

So put bluntly it takes your testosterone and turns it into estrogen. It takes what makes you're a man and turns it into what makes one a woman. Think about that. So obviously this is something that we really want to take care of and make sure is addressed.

One of the biggest and most problematic sources of aromatase in your body is extra fat. Meaning pretty much any fat above ten to fifteen percent body fat. Especially fat that is centered around the gut area. You want to get rid of this fat so that you will be getting rid of the aromatase that converts testosterone into estrogen. You also want to make sure that you are getting adequate zinc in your diet which helps with estrogen and aromatase. Another thing that is great for taking care of excess estrogen and aromatase is cruciferous vegetables (think broccoli). Also obviously avoid toxic weakening agents such as soy and soy's big brother alcohol. Remember that soy is in pretty much every non organic product including animal meats.

Insulin

Alright now it's time for some myth busting. So insulin regulated your blood sugar but this is why you care about it. When insulin goes up testosterone goes down and there is a direct correlation between people who are insulin resistant and low testosterone levels. Here is what causes insulin sugar and carbs. So when you eat a lot of carbs you get a lot of insulin spikes and when you get a lot of insulin spikes you get fat and insulin resistant. I'm over simplifying but you get the general idea. Now obviously all carbs are not created the same. Both broccoli and candy bars are considered carbs. To have high testosterone you want to avoid all carbs that aren't vegetables. You want to avoid things that contain sugars or grains. Nothing new here but as an added bonus will also help with your testosterone.

You want to avoid things like orange juice, cakes, breads, and all other assorted foods. It if it's high in sugar or grain or starch then you don't want it. The more you tend towards a paleo/keto esque (no diet is perfect, use common sense) type of diet the better off that you'll be. If you are insulin resistant you want to remedy this ASAP. Consume good fats (especially omega-3 like fish oil) and get your body fat down (those two things work synergistically). Adding in some high rep squats, barbell complexes, or sprints will all help in getting body fat down as well as have a host of other positive T boosting effects. So for peak testosterone stay away from the vast majority of carbs. Unless it's green and a vegetable it's most likely not going to be good for your testosterone levels. Insulin resistance is an enemy of testosterone. Keep it in check.

Summary

Alright so a lot of what's here goes against many of what is said both by bros and clowns in lab coats who don't know the first thing about testosterone. But more importantly these things work. When you understand the principles of raising testosterone (and what creates it) you understand what to do to have peak testosterone. Focus on principles which are much more important than methods/details. For example say I know the effects insulin has but then read a study about these doctors that tested three rats giving them carbs of wheat bread and their testosterone raised by 25% does that mean I'd run out an start eating bread by the loaf? Of course not, because I understand the principle which is more important than some random study. Not to mention the millions of variables that could have taken place. From who sponsored the study to the beliefs of the doctors to a million other things.

There are a million reasons why studies are ineffective at best. People who rely on them completely have no mind of their own and cannot see what's in front of them. Principles over details. Use your own mind and brain don't slavishly follow dubious methods and sources. Like I've said men knew deep down that things like bacon, eggs, and steak were good for them even when all the doctors, studies, and media said they weren't. Use your own mind and brain and understand the principles which are what is important. This applies to all fields not just health and testosterone optimization. Use your own mind and look for similarities between principles.

The Most Important Macronutrient For Optimal Testosterone Production

Not all macronutrients are created equal. There are three types of macronutrients that we are all familiar with they are as follows fats, proteins, and carbohydrates. Much has been written about each and they are all important to learn about for maximal functioning of your body. From hormonal health to body composition to energy levels to overall health. Micronutrients are things like zinc, potassium, and vitamin K. Which are also important but have been covered in other areas as far as optimizing testosterone goes. Like I've said never forget that a base line of health will help in all that you are trying to do. For example losing body fat will not only help with how good you look but also increase your testosterone levels as well as give you more energy.

Like good habits good health has a cumulative effect. Alright so now let's get down to the macronutrients.

So much has been written about all three macronutrients before. Right now there is a hot debate going on about carbohydrates some say that they are the devil incarnate while others say you can build muscle or live a healthy life without them. One who has no idea what they are talking about will always say "the truth lies somewhere in the middle" or some other B.S. While both statements are false the truth does not lie somewhere in the middle and rarely ever does. Here we are going to go through a breakdown of the three macronutrients and how they relate to hormonal optimization and in particular increasing testosterone levels as high as possible.

Carbohydrates & Protein

Alright we're going to address carbohydrates and proteins first. Both are important for optimized health and both are important for body composition. And both can play a role in testosterone production and optimization albeit not directly. We'll start with protein. If you've been around body building or fitness circles for any length of time then you've probably heard that as far as macronutrients go protein is the holy grail. While protein is certainly important getting in huge quantities of it isn't going to do that much for your overall health, hormone optimization, or even muscle building. I used to eat one gram per pound and have found that to be way too high.

Now I eat much less but my body composition hasn't changed. If you're eating lots of meats, eggs, and good dairy each day then you don't have to worry too much about protein. Too much protein won't kill you or anything it just isn't optimal and a waste. There comes a point where eating more protein won't do much for you. As long as you're getting somewhere around a gram per pound of lean body mass (and the source matters a ton too, such as a steak is one hundred times better than a powder) you'll be fine.

Anything above that takes away from other sources of nutrients.

Now for carbohydrates. First off carbohydrates are not needed for building muscle. Carbohydrates such as anything processed, grains, and starchy carbs aren't good for you and should be removed from your diet. Not only do they spike insulin and cause insulin resistance. Which leads to higher body fat and lower testosterone but there are also a host of other negative effects that they have on the body that entire books have been written about. As far as carbohydrates go you want to make sure you're getting them from sources such as sweet potatoes and green vegetables. All carbs are not created equal. And anyone who talks about carbs as a group making blanket statements such as "carbs increase testosterone" need to dive deeper. For example broccoli can increase testosterone levels while a potato or something made from wheat bread will cause insulin spikes that will lower testosterone. Stick to greens for optimized hormones when it comes to carbohydrates.

Fats

Alright now here is where we are getting into what really makes for great hormonal health and high levels of testosterone. Put simply (as there are many body processes that take part in producing testosterone from the brain to the balls literally) testosterone comes from cholesterol (as well as a host of other hormones). Meaning that the macronutrient that is most important to optimized hormonal levels and in particular maximizing how much testosterone your body produces is fat. In particular saturated fat and cholesterol, you know the stuff that our benevolent protectors at the government and medical establishment have told us is straight up poison for the last twenty or more years. Yeah that stuff.

You want to eat things like grass fed beef, bacon, and free range eggs. Things that have good saturated fats (that are essential for testosterone production) as well as cholesterol (again essential for testosterone production). Fats are by far the most important macronutrient for hormone optimization and testosterone production. Especially saturated fats and cholesterol. Now like carbs (and protein, aka powder vs meat) not all fats are created equal. Trans fats and even high levels of polysaturated fats (omega-6 not omega-3) lower testosterone. So avoid vegetable oils (olives are a fruit) and fats from processed foods which lower testosterone. Eat lots of good saturated fats and cholesterol. Doing this will optimize your hormones and testosterone production.

Other Things To Avoid

Obviously there are many other things to avoid and take care of but you already know that. I'll high light a couple things here as both a refresher and to include some new things I haven't hit on as much as I would have liked too. Alright so one of the number one things that can wreak havoc not just with your overall health but your testosterone production as well (as the two are tied together) is sugar. One of the reason that low carb diets work so well (in addition to getting rid of grains which have much of the same effect as sugar sometimes even stronger) is because of the elimination of sugar from the diet and elimination of things that work like sugar. For example bread spikes your insulin level in much the same way as sugar (including "healthy" whole grain bread).

Another thing about sugar is that it depletes other micronutrients (also very important for hormonal health and testosterone production) for example potassium which most people don't get enough of anyways. Now like everything else not all sugars are created equal. For example pure natural Tupelo honey isn't nearly as bad for you as pure white sugar that you'll find in all different kinds of food. Of course it's still sugar it just isn't going to have as much as a negative effect as the pure white stuff. For the most part you are going to want to avoid sugar especially processed sugar. This may be tough to kick but anyone who told you optimizing hormones, health, and testosterone levels was easy is a liar. You are going to have to change your lifestyle. It's not easy but it is more than worth it. I should also note that alcohol (including wine or whatever drink you've rationalized is good for you) has much of the same negative effects, get rid of it.

Summary

So all macronutrients play a role on overall health, hormonal health, and testosterone optimization however by far the most important is fat in particular saturated fat and cholesterol. So make sure you're cooking up lots of eggs (even though eating them raw is how you get the most nutrients from them) as well as bacon, beef, and other true "super foods". Not all proteins, carbs, or fats are created equal so it's hard to make blanket statements about each without clarifying. For example green vegetables (a carb) are awesome for hormonal health and testosterone production meanwhile grains and sugars (also carbs) are killers for testosterone and overall health. So make sure that you read the fine print when looking into all of this stuff. So now go out and eats lot of saturated fats and cholesterol from good sources and become more of a man.

3 Foods Men Need To Eat More Of

If you look at the modern male's diet it's a wreck. Either it's tampon flavored tofu and pesticide free lettuce or it's beer and carbs. Neither is going to result in anything good. Health is one part of your life that you don't want to neglect. You can be wealthy with all the buxom beautiful babes in the world and one heart attack could end it all. You have to keep your health in working order. Take your health seriously and you'll have a higher standard of living than the vast majority.

Most people just simply drift through life just going whatever which way to current of the world takes them. They just hope a good woman will fall in their lap, strong fighting muscles will be theirs, and that money will rain down on them suddenly one day. Most people leave their fate up to luck and chance. Which if you know anything about the world you know is beyond foolish. People need guidance to get anything they want in life, they need right direction. This chapter here is a step in the right direction for the diets of the modern Western male.

Food #1 – Steak

The king of food. Men don't eat enough steak. Unless you're eating this great food multiple times a week you are not getting enough of it. Steak contains lots of protein as well as fats needed for proper hormone production (aka testosterone production). Anyone who tells you that steak/red meat is bad for you wants you to be weak and testosterone free. Steak also contains zinc which is critical to adequate testosterone production not to mention keeping your immune system strong.

So essentially eating steak makes you strong, manly, and disease free exactly the opposite of how the government wants you. No wonder there have been so many campaigns to associate steak with being unhealthy while pushing estrogen raising and gut expanding foods. Steak should be a staple of your diet. While it can run expensive there are a variety of cuts as well as prep methods to keep things fresh and not too expensive.

Food #2 – Eggs

Another food that has been maligned and told was bad for us by those caring individuals of the U.S. government and medical establishment. Eggs have many of the same effects as steak. Namely making you strong, manly, and healthy. Eggs also contain good amounts of protein and fat and are much cheaper than steak (though not a replacement). Make sure you are eating both the white and the yolk. The yolk contains much needed fats that are critical in hormone production (aka testosterone).

You wouldn't throw testosterone down the drain so don't throw the egg yolks down the drain either. All parts of the egg are good for you. The white contains large amounts of protein and the yolks contain needed fats as well as have a variety of nutrients in them as well. Nutrients such as vitamins A, E, & D for starters. Which covers everything from your mood to your immune system. Eat lots of eggs often.

Food #3 – Cheese

While most males who are aware of their health and the reality of nutrition know that steak and eggs are good for them, some forget to consider another great food. Cheese is another great food that men need to eat more off. Cheese like steak and eggs also contains protein, though not as quite as high of amount. It also contains good nutrients that are required for hormone development as well as generally costs less than steak and is on par with eggs.

There are many different types of cheese and they are not created equal. Obviously I'm not talking about the cheese you'll find on your burger at McDonalds nor the kind that comes in a can. Cheese like American, cheddar, Munster, provolone, goat, etc. In addition to having protein cheese also contains saturated fat which is needed for optimal testosterone production as well as feelings of well-being. Include cheese as a staple of your diet in addition to steak and eggs.

Summary

You'll notice some similarities from all the foods above. Namely they contain high amounts of protein and saturated fat. Two very important things and two things that in a large part make a man a man. You'll also notice that whenever something makes a man strong, manly, and healthy the government and medical establishment will come out against it declaring that it is bad for you. For good health ignore the government, the medical establishment, as well as the hordes of sheeple being led to the slaughter. Do your own research and figure out what's best for you. You'll find that the three foods above will always be a staple of any sane diet for men.

A Cheat Sheet For Increasing Your Testosterone

Alright so I've written a lot about optimizing your hormones and raising your testosterone as high as it can be naturally. However there is a lot of information and it can be overwhelming at times. So what I'm going to do here is give you a cheat sheet meaning a simplified breakdown of all the actionable steps that you should be taking and in the correct order of importance. Optimizing testosterone just like getting in shape whether you're trying to build big muscles, get rid of fat, or both can be very complicated when you're thrown information (even if it's great information) from every different direction. So it's good to have something that focuses everything that we have learned and allows us to make the most out of it.

I also want to point out while some things are certainly more important than others, for example getting enough sleep is far more important than whether you take your ZMA or not, that everything still works together. Meaning that everything feeds into each other. Becoming healthier in one area is going to help you in others making for a positive loop, something I talk a lot about in The Primer and would recommend you check out to learn more. So for example eating healthier will give your body the energy that it needs to hit the gym harder which translates into better sleep and so on and so forth. Not to mention all of those things also contribute to hormonal health and testosterone optimization. Everything is connected, especially when it comes to your health. Alright now for the cheat sheet for increasing your testosterone.

Level 1 – Sleep

Without sleep you won't be producing any testosterone. You

could have a perfect diet, train like a beast, as well as be free of any environmental hormonal disruptors yet without sleep you're not going to have high levels of testosterone, simple as that. Make sure that you're getting around 8-9 hours if not more. If you must be in bed before ten to make sure that you have plenty of time to sleep. Many people see sleep as something that gets in the way of productivity and therefore do not place much importance on it, this is a mistake to put it lightly. Sleep is incredibly important of health at all levels, and your hormones and testosterone production is no exception. Don't neglect this vital part of your life.

Do everything you can to maximize the quality of your sleep as well. If that means spending some extra money to get a nicer mattress, placing fans strategically around your bed (a must for me), and getting black out shades then do so. There are plenty of things that you spend money and time optimizing that are not one one hundredth as important as the sleep that you get. Put priority on this and your body (and testosterone) will thank you. Experiment with different things to see how they affect your sleep, like with anything else take what works for you and discard what doesn't. But regardless make sure to give sleep the importance that it deserves.

Level 2 – Nutrition

After sleep the next most important thing is nutrition. Without proper nutrition you're not going to make testosterone in healthy amounts. Most people eat a crap diet, no surprise there but even many who are eating "healthy" without injecting testosterone can be killing their testosterone levels with their diet. Many common diets even ones that may be good for overall body composition are not great for hormones. Also as a side note getting below ten percent body fat also negatively effects testosterone. There is a marked difference between one whose hormones are optimized and one whose body is optimized to impress judges at a bodybuilding contest or photo shoot. Try to stick between 12-15% body fat otherwise your libido and testosterone production are going to take a dive.

Alright for hormonal optimization you want to make sure that you are getting as much food as you can from natural sources meaning that pretty much anything from a farmer's market is going to be better for you than something from a big box store (or even a specialty "health" store). Avoiding pesticides and other crap is a must. It can be expensive but you're better off eating less good food then you are eating more processed and modified foods. For a general recommendation about eating for hormonal optimization you want to eat lots of fats and avoid most carbs (other than vegetables). Think paleo or keto type diets. You don't have to follow them exactly just trying to give you an overall general idea of the type of foods and diet structure you want. High fats, moderate protein, and for the most part low carbs (can raise carbs on training days if needed).

Level 3 – Training

For hormonal health pretty much any kind of resistance training is going to help improve it and increase testosterone levels. However not all methods are created equal. Also you want to make sure to avoid things like long distance running or triathlon type training which will crush testosterone levels. You want relatively short intense bursts of activity. You want your workouts to be under an hour and you want to go heavy, hit it hard, then get out. You want to focus on full body workouts and compound movements. You want to hit everything and hit it fast, so things like squats and deadlifts are going to do more than cable work or isolation work will ever do as far as hormonal health goes.

Here are some examples of good testosterone producing workouts. Something like Bill Starr's 5×5 where you're doing a heavy push, pull, and squat three times a week. I also like things like barbell complexes, sprints, and high rep squats as they all have a large hormonal impact on the body and follow the principles of working out for hormonal health (namely intense compound movements). Do what works for you if that's full body workouts three times a week then do that. If that's something different but uses those movements above and has high intensity then do that. Just make sure you're not spending hours in the gym doing isolation exercises or jogging for hours. Put simply workout like a man.

Level 4 – Environment

The third level is taking care of your environment. This means avoiding as much chemicals and other hormone destroying things as you can. Some simple steps to do this are eating organic food (covered in the nutrition section), switching from plastic glasses and containers to glass, and staying away from as many man-made chemicals as you can. This can also mean switching from main steam personal care products to ones that are more naturally produced and don't contain the harmful testosterone sapping chemicals that main stream ones do. For example anything that contains parabens in it can hurt your testosterone levels and anything containing BPA can absolutely wreck your hormonal health and in particular your testosterone production.

The biggest source of BPA is plastic water bottles so make sure to get rid of those ASAP. You also want to make sure you're using a water filter because tap water is filled with fluoride which also lowers testosterone. In addition to all this you want to manage your stress as best as possible. Fortunately things like sleep, nutrition, and training will all help with this. But if you need to include meditation or listening to classical music at the end of the day to take off the edge then do that as well. Do what works for you to keep stress low. I try as hard as I can to make sure that my overall stress levels are kept low as possibly but that's not always possible and I have found walks in nature does wonders for me. Do what works for you.

Level 5 – Supplementation

This is by far the least important part of the process. Don't get me wrong supplementation certainly helps and can work wonders especially when you are deficient in certain vitamins and minerals (which the vast majority of men are). The two prime ones that help tremendously in testosterone production and most men are deficient in are zinc and vitamin D (which is actually a steroidal hormone). Magnesium also helps. This is why the only testosterone boosting supplements that I recommend are ZMA and vitamin D. Fish oil also can help through helping with insulin so I take that as well but that is for general health reasons and all the benefits that fish oil provides.

Regardless you should strive to get all the macro and micronutrients that you need from real food sources.

But in reality that isn't always possible so it's good to have supplements to take up the slack. They aren't going to completely turn your testosterone levels around but they certainly help and are worth the investment. Just understand what place in the hierarchy that they occupy. Don't worry about what brand of ZMA you're getting if you're sleeping on a mattress that isn't comfortable or you're sweating when trying to fall asleep at night. Take care of the important things first and then take care of the least important things. Makes sense but few do it, those that do though are the ones that get the most from it.

Again obvious but something to keep in mind.

Summary

Alright so I'll give you a quick breakdown of what you need to do to optimize testosterone. This is made to be a quick reference list. Don't skip everything read this list only and then complain if things don't work. It's important to know the why behind things so that you can adjust them as needed and see if they apply to you. Blindly following a cookie cutter program of any sort will generally not get you the results that you want, always learn the why behind things. Now with that being said here are the actionable items that you can implement right away to get your testosterone levels optimized naturally.

Get 8-9 hours of sleep. Eat enough good fats, adequate protein, and in general keep your carbs low (get most if not all of your carbs from green vegetables). Training like a man. Lift heavy shit for short periods of time, do sprints, squat, you get the general idea. Get rid of as many chemicals as you can. Drink from glass, don't microwave food in plastic containers, avoid processed foods. Cut out as much stress as possible, do meditation or nature walks if you want. Take ZMA and vitamin D. There you have it do these things and you'll be on your way to hormonal optimization, feeling great, and high levels of testosterone. Now get to it.

About The Author

Enjoyed the content? Then could you do me a favor? Leave a review on Amazon or tell a friend about the ways that the book has helped you. I love reading how my books have positively affected the lives of my readers. I read each and every review, they mean a lot to me. If you want to learn more I run a blog at charlessledge.com where you can find more content to further your masculine development to new heights. If you found value in the book drop by and join the community. Looking forward to hearing from you.

-Charles Sledge

Made in the USA
Middletown, DE
25 January 2019